Dedicated to an everlasting role model

M.D. Tophus

Attitudinal and Personality Traits in the Individual and Healthcare.

Hilphma Publications 2023. www.hilphmapublication.com

First Edition.

Germany.

The author has over 25 years of clinical experience in the healthcare field. Is cognisant of both DSM-5-TR (and previous versions) and ICD-11 (and previous versions) disorders and conditions; quality and safety improvement in healthcare; and healthcare education

Other M.D. Tophus publications available:

"Exercising Quality in Healthcare Service Provision: A Complex Care Workbook for All Healthcare Professionals." Germany: Hilphma Publications: 2022.

"Who is This Colleague?: Dangers of the Healthcare Profession, and beyond. An Interview Guide for Recruitment, Performance Appraisal and Post-Adverse Events."
Germany: Hilphma Publications: 2022.

"Think on your Feet: Those Who Can. For the Consummate Healthcare Professional."
Germany: Hilphma Publications: 2022.

"The Unfortunate Healthcare Treater, The Hapless Healthcare Therapist: Narcissistic and Borderline Personality Disorder clients. The Grit."
Germany: Hilphma Publications: 2022.

"Victims of Crime: Introduction to Forensic Challenges in Healthcare."
Germany: Hilphma Publications: 2022.

"The A to Z of Workplace Bullying: For the Healthcare Professional and Beyond."
Germany: Hilphma Publications: 2022.

"Trauma United, Life Defined. A Healthcare Tool for Professionals Across the Globe."
Germany: Hilphma Publications: 2022.

"Reflective Thinking: the True Healthcare Tool."
Germany: Hilphma Publications: 2022.

"Burnout in Healthcare"
Germany: Hilphma Publications: 2022.

"Reasonable Resilience in Workplaces and Healthcare Work"
Germany: Hilphma Publications: 2022.

"The Psychological Impacts of Labelling and Failure to Diagnose".
Germany: Hilphma Publications: 2022.

"The Controversy of the Remorseless and Unempathic Healthcare Worker"
Germany: Hilphma Publications: 2023.

CONTENTS

Attitudinal traits are an essentiality to personality traits. Without an understanding of personality traits emerges erasure of attitudinal traits and their importance.

Personality traits inspire several functional elements which cannot be erased due to era, modernisation, or nouveau psychological reasoning.

Essential personality traits can include birth to death traits; unique adjustment to one's environment; conscious and unconscious motivations of thought; childhood experiences; and, openness to experience; conscientiousness; agreeableness; extroversion; and emotional stability.

Attitudunal traits, although potentially influenced by training and education, are an exposé of an individual's inner self, feelings, emotions, emotional responses, and resultant behavioral counterparts. They are more than a complimentary addition to personality traits, they are indomitably representative of personality traits, in the main.

This relates, highly, to patient quality and safety.

The battle between inner self and societal attitudes remains true.

Thus, ethical dilemmas, and alternatively- ethically damaging conceptualisations, are at the forefront of loggerheads- in the mainstream.

In addition, healthcare and its magnanimous efforts to overcome pressures from socio-politico-forces, and to utilise the inner workings of each and every healthcare worker's ethico-psychological commitments, are often hindered by the modern day push for social self- and the idea that personality traits and attitudes can vacillate according to ever-changing psycho-social norms.

This publication incorporates inner self, core personality traits, and attitudinal traits, examination of ethical stances, personality assessment, traits and expectations of healthcare workers, personality disorders, and developmental psychology, which is relevant for all walks of life.
It includes healthcare in the main, and analysis of healthcare workers' attitudes.
It is written from a psychological perspective, but integrates sociological understandings.
A comprehensive set of test questions, is inclusive.

<u>INNER SELF</u>

As simple as it appears, it is highly challenging to provide intersectional differentiation (in-sectional explanatories), in relation to the 'inner self'.
Thus, due to the integrated nature of the inner self, several of the sections' entries are, at times, interrelated.

*The **<u>inner self</u>** (usually) comprises the following essentials (and more):*

personal values

-core beliefs adhered to by which one lives their life

-morality, including conceptualisations between right and wrong decisions and behaviors

-ethical principles

-priorities

-ideals

It has been suggested that there are <u>10 basic human values</u>:

-self-direction;

-stimulation;

-hedonism;

-achievement;

-power;

-security;

-conformity;

-tradition;

-benevolence;

-universalism.

(1)

intuition

-reliance on one's own inner sense

-instinctive versus conscious reasoning which is synonymous with knowledge, feeling, and
 understanding

-beyond thinking, reflecting, and rationalizing.

beliefs

This involves:

-sub-conscious,

-non-conscious, and

-conscious

cognitive processes.

Furthermore, belief in self is enhanced by one's ability to:

-attain and utilise knowledge, experience, and intuition, effectively

-facilitate a more cogent belief system used with confidence and consistency.

This positively effects accurate decision making.

personality characteristics

Integral to one's personality characteristics, are:

-abilities

-primary traits

-both psychologically, and biologically, affected

-represented by one's thoughts, emotions, feelings and behaviors, which effects

  choice, mode, and frequency of:

  -social interaction;

-choice and pursuit of interests;

-level of hopefulness

-degree of contentment

 -innate self-regulation

-choice of coping strategies

-work conduct, attitude, and productivity

and much more.

feelings/emotional responses, content

Though feelings and emotional responses can be enhanced by specific locations, and contributing factors related to environment, the following are examples of importance to the inner self:

-capacity for empathy

-emotional reactions to fear and anger

-level of sadness, happiness.

Where there is a satisfactory (or more) amount of self-awareness regarding emotional responses and feelings- which encapsulate the inner self- emotional content is more easily recognised.

immediate inner reactions to people, environments, circumstances
(including challenges)

-exposure to one's inner self is often more tangible when one is faced with a challenge

-whether the challenge be due to a conflict, plans which have gone awry, or some form of heartbreak, often one is left to cope independently

-experience of a challenge/s in life and ones which cause you to question yourself, your capabilities, and your intuitive processes, elicit untamed responses to people, environments and circumstances

-this is not necessarily a negative situation, as it facilitates greater knowledge of oneself's inner workings.

identity

Knowledge of:

-your purpose in life,

-your likes,

-passions and

-dislikes,

without being influenced by others.

self-awareness

Capacity to understand the effects that you have:

-on others,

-your environments, and

-the world around you.

A comprehension of your own values, and reasons for being motivated to reflect, to behave in a certain way, or your immediate, innate reactions to specific circumstances, are inclusive of self-awareness.

the true self

-embraces the concept of me, myself, and I

-the true self often differs from one's social self

-an assured presence of mind and behavior can access the truth about oneself, along with other inner self attributes.

vulnerabilities

-idiosyncracies

-fears

-self-protective (defensive) thoughts and behaviors

-intolerances

-at-risk thoughts and behaviors

are part of each individual's makeup.

self-esteem

Self-esteem can be influenced by childhood experiences, lifestyle, and significant relationships. All these factors can singularly, or in combination, affect the inner workings of one's self.

The propensity for a healthy (moderate to high level of), or not so healthy, degree of self-esteem is influenced by the following:

-level of confidence (relates to self-confidence) in one's capabilities and qualities

-coherency of/realistic levels of: belief in achieving goals, objectives, and life plans

-self-respect

-self-trust

-worthiness of self (to self)

-ability (or inability) to temper ongoing, or generalised, self-criticism

-propensity for recognition of when appropriate assertive thought, action and behavior, is of necessity

-understanding of the differences between ideal self and real self.

Your values, attitudes, and beliefs, contribute to self-knowledge of your primary aims, and behaviors.

'Personal values' (as abovementioned) are consistent with this, including that of ethical principles.

-"The individual (personal) level of the self-concept focusses on unique individual traits, abilities, and goals"
(2)

The entries included in: 'identity'; 'self-awareness'; 'the true self'; and, 'self-esteem', are highly consistent with this section.

For those subscribing to humanist and existential psychological themes,

-self-actualisation is considered the pinnacle of achievement in self-growth, particularly as featured in Maslow's hierarchy of needs.

- Rogers also esteemed self-actualization as indicative of optimal functioning along with unconditional acceptance, and love.

self-belief

Though connected to self-confidence, 'self-belief' incorporates a wider variety of variables, such as, that:

-one has enough self-value to utilise their core attributes, and qualities

-deep conceptualisations of success in achieving, completing, or furthering of, one's highly held innate principles

-under duress, your inner self will remain intact

-upon external forces (or persons) challenging your self-confidence based thoughts and behaviors, that your identity, principles, ethics, and related thoughts and actions, will prevail

-likewise, with attempted destruction of one's self-confidence, the inner person will continue to exist.

effective utilisation of intelligence

This is substantially connected to the concept of 'intuition', and is explicated by way of:

-mental fitness to undertake clear cognitions, and decision-making

-involving an inner self- connected assessment of one's self- to ascertain accurately
 perceptive judgements, and abilities

-emotional intelligence as part of the 'utilisation of intelligence' process.

creativity

-inventive abilities which enact the principles of the inner self

-problem solving abilities realised

-examination of alternative options

-inception of different ideas, and concepts.

self-efficacy

-is task specific

-dovetails with self-belief, and self-regulation, processes

-involves confidence and belief in self regarding task performance abilities

-true confidence in one's own capacity to reach and achieve goals and objectives

-this also involves motivation to continue working consistently to reach goals; and the
ability to affect change

-this covers the full spectrum of life, including that of work related tasks such as clinical
decision-making

-however, it does involve self-compassion.

capacity to have hopes and dreams (and attempted realisation, thereof)

Psyche based contributions realise one's inner self (thoughts, emotions, actions and behaviors) to actualise their realistic potential along with advancing their future prospects.

that no two people are exactly alike

-one can compliment the other

-or on the other hand have the ability to

    -coerce,

    -influence, or

    -cajole

into changing another individual's focus upon what is important, or valuable in life

-however, an exact true replica of another individual can never exist.

Nevertheless the inner core, regardless of if it is perceived as irreparable, intangible, or destroyed, remains (though perhaps perceptually hidden) throughout one's lifetime.

CORE PERSONALITY TRAITS

Historical relevance:

Historically vital, Allport's definition of personality is: of primary uniqueness within an individual.

He categorised personality traits into:

- **cardinal traits** (rare in persons, normally develop in latter life, and, is a determinant of behavior. In addition to self-sacrificial leanings, this can also include: greed, ambition, and compulsive lying)

- **central traits** (core but do not 'determine' behaviors)

- **secondary traits** (reliant on immediate situation and context).

His last publication emphasised cognitive processes (conscious planning and 'intentions') more.

He also emphasised the important influence of conscious motivations and thoughts.

Additionally, that:

-problems in childhood (whereby needs were unmet), thence, in adulthood,- one can become stuck at childhood phase/s of development

-the psycho-physical in personality creates 'unique adjustment' to his/her environment.

He was a critic of Freud and his focus was on the unconscious (but believed in unconscious memory).

Integral with this, is the:

-pro- understanding of the individual, and against authoritarianism in psychology

-exemplified by: *"An attitude is a state of mental and neural readiness, organized through experience, exerting a directive or dynamic influence upon the individual's response to all objects and situations with which it is related"*
(3)

<u>**Examination of Prejudice:**</u>

Allport thoroughly examined the concept of prejudice, including determining that:

-personality is determined at birth (biological)

-childhood experiences, and current environment, and interaction, between each helps create influences upon personality

-religion, whereby he developed the 'religious orientation scale'/questionnaire- of two dimensions-, is categorised into: intrinsic (deep/mature faith determining way of life type, ego and those believing in religion as primary motive involving influence upon interpretation of life and life events); and, extrinsic (immature faith, self-serving)

-and, was pro-study of religious meaning to an individual versus comparing religious faith between people.

Interestingly, his perspective regarding his very much focussed upon topic of religion, was essentially:

"...seeking to trace the full course of religious development in the normally mature and productive personality. I am dealing with the psychology, not with the psychopathology of religion....Many personalities attain a religious view of life without suffering arrested development and without self-deception". (4)

Again, as with personality, faith experienced/held by an individual is non-identical to each other, it is individual.

He placed much focus on prejudice and religion (that is, attitudes and religion).

For instance, in reference to immature (extrinsic versus intrinsic) faith:

"Immature religion, whether in adult or child, is largely concerned with magical thinking, self-justification, and creature comfort. Thus it betrays its sustaining motives still to be the drives and desires of the body." (5)

His personality traits' work invariably contributed to research which inspired formulation of the FFM (five factor model) of personality. (6)

The FFM (Five factor model) of personality traits includes (often referred to as) OCEAN: Openness to Experience; Conscientiousness; Extraversion; Agreeableness; Neuroticism.

The HEXACO model, though it incorporates the Five Factors, also includes:

-honesty-humility as a 6th factor- a vital quality, especially in the healthcare arena

-use of 'emotionality' instead of neuroticism (sometimes referred to as Emotional Stability/Instability)

-'agreeableness (versus anger)' is used instead of 'agreeableness'. (7)

The 6 factors (+ 1 interstitial) are explained below (via scales):

Openness to Experience: **Aesthetic Appreciation; Inquisitiveness; Creativity; Unconventionality**

-aesthetic appreciation: enjoyment of nature and artistic endeavours

-inquisitiveness: curiosity, for instance, about intellectual pursuits

-creativity: innovative approaches to problem-solving, and have an artistic focus

-unconventionality: expanding thoughts to include alternative views.

Conscientiousness: **Organization; Diligence; Perfectionism; Prudence**

-organization: ordered occupational, and other areas of life

-diligence: hard workers

-perfectionism: thorough, with attention to detail

-prudence: non-impulsive cognitions and behaviors.

Extraversion: **Social Self-Esteem; Social Boldness; Sociability; Liveliness**

-social self-esteem: confident in interacting, in a variety of social situations

-social boldness: enjoys socialising, and being the focus of attention

-sociability: enthusiastic upon thoughts of, or when, socialising

-liveliness: energetic and positive disposition.

Agreeableness (versus Anger): **Forgivingness; Gentleness; Flexibility; Patience**

-forgivingness: ability to let hurts go

-gentleness: minimal judgement of others

-flexibility: co-operative with the capacity to undertake compromise

-patience: tempered negative emotions even in the case of others displaying them.

Emotionality:
Fearfulness; Anxiety; Dependence; Sentimentality

-fearfulness: reduced anxiety regarding life stressors

-anxiety: worry about bigger versus smaller issues, fear (of for instance, physical endangerment)

-dependence: requirement of emotional support not necessary unless faced with a major stressor

-sentimentality: capacity for empathy and emotional connection with others

are inclusive.

Honesty- Humility:

Sincerity; Fairness; Greed Avoidance; Modesty

Cogent to this category, are:

-manipulation (sincerity)

-rule breaking (fairness)

- focus on wealth (greed avoidance)

- high social status (modesty).

Naturally, upon testing, a person with high scores on this domain, will have low to nil levels of manipulation, and so forth.

There is also an 'interstitial' scale: Altruism (versus Antagonism).

Contrasting with the above model, are the Dark triad personality traits (8):

The core traits are featured below, but several listed can be interchangeable with the other dark triad personality traits described.

Machiavellianism:

-nil empathy

-highly manipulative

-deceitful

-liars

-tricksters

-cunning

-selfish

-morally corrupt

-cheaters

-act completely in their own self-interests

-exploitative

-highly competitive

-extremely ambitious

-seek power at all costs

all behaviors are often masked by charm.

Narcissism:

-lack of empathy (especially in malignant narcissism)

-highly manipulative

-proud

-ego driven

-entitled

-grandiose

-superior

-self-important

-liars

-dominant

often masked by charm.

<u>Psychopathy:</u>

-nil empathy

-high level of impulsivity

-highly manipulative

-liars

-selfish

-callous

-anti-social behaviors

-risky behaviors

-callous disregard

-ruthlessness

to get what 'they' want, often masked by charm.

With further relevance, are the DSM-5-TR personality trait domains (and their polar opposites) are:

Negativity (versus Emotional Stability); Detachment (versus Extraversion); Antagonism (versus Agreeableness); Disinhibition (versus Conscientiousness); and, Psychoticism (versus Lucidity). (9)

ATTITUDINAL TRAITS

It is argued that trait influences upon attitudes involve:

self-confidence, self-esteem, self-efficacy, connected classifications- along with the five factor personality traits.

Attitudinal traits involve:

Cognitive: thoughts and beliefs.

Affective: emotional response to person, circumstance or object.

Behavioral: how attitudes define actions.

They also incorporate: implicit and explicit biases/attitudes.

Change:

They can be cultivated by training and education.

-However, core attitudinal traits (as linked with personality traits) are very difficult to change.

Change is ripe, where there exists:

-lack of self-identity,

-low level moral stage of development, and

-submissiveness.

Modes of Change:

Modes of change which contribute to some attitudinal traits, include:

-observation

-behavioral conditioning

-social self

-modelled behaviors can influence many of one's attitudes, however- the inner self, and the extent to which one knows oneself, are the predominating features defining attitudinal traits.

Opinions (externalised, or less meaningful to one's true self) differ, they remain part of attitudes one holds, but can be altered or changed.

Influences (Resistance and Compliance):

A person's level of:

-determination

-stubborness

-identification with refusal to be attitudinally shifted by others

-circumstances

-challenges

become important in influencing (or not), attitudinally.

So, too:

-past experiences of indoctrination

-experiences of subterfuge (where lies may have been told to change one's attitudinal position)

-social self, and compliance with norms defined by the social circle/environment

-alternatively, a firm commitment to fully investigating and educating oneself on each factor involved before decision making about a subject, person, or circumstance,

are also factors.

<u>**Personality types:**</u>

Cognition and affect relate directly to one's personality traits.

For instance, an extrovert will not necessarily value depth of thought and insight before reacting to an immediate situation in the same way that an introvert may.

Likewise, a person who is less conscientious is potentially prone to responding with a given (perhaps, negative) emotion when a stressor is presented before them.

<u>**Compromising attitudinal traits:**</u>

The *Five Hazardous Attitudes* (10) are:

Anti-authority: 'don't tell me'

Impulsivity: 'do it quick'

Invulnerability: 'it won't happen to me'

Macho: 'I can do it'

Resignation: 'What's the use?'

<u>**Relevance to Healthcare:**</u>

This can directly cross-reference to other work environments involving high risk, and life and death situations- especially that of healthcare. Likewise, examination of threats to safety and quality, near misses, accidents, undertaking root cause analysis, action following learnings from analysing what occurred; productive assistance in reduction of medical errors: can, and have been, applied to healthcare environments.

How this relates to attitudinal and personality traits is a given, as in the exemplifications provided formerly.

Helpful mechanisms such as- root cause analysis (to re-iterate)- can facilitate identification of attitudinal traits, in particular, ones which are of perilous existence within the healthcare industry.

Arguably, and formulaically, this (from a worker's perspective, respectfully) is presented as such:

innate traits + childhood experiences + current situation/ circumstances/environment + apathy + burnout+ meaninglessness + questioning of career, ambitions, goals, objectives + dislike of work + dislike of work environment, colleagues + duties--> interventionist supportive leadership enhancing versus changing the worker--> aggregated enhancement of self + aim for higher self/ self-actualisation (in a graspable/ tangible way) + celebration of uniqueness and personality traits

ETHICAL STANCES

Value of ethics:

-emanating from the inner core/self,

-utilised with intuitive cognitive processes,

-plus life experiences,

develops value (or not) of ethics and utilisation in life and at work.

It very much depends upon stage of moral development; and, the level of importance (and understanding) placed upon:

-right versus wrong; and

-capacity for empathic feeling.

Innate leaning toward ethics:

Past experiences (value placed upon vicarious learning), or witnessing of:

-conceptualised and recognised injustices

-dangers (including errors and risks involved in quality of healthcare and patient safety)

all effect an innate leaning toward:

   -actualising the use of ethics

-facing ethical dilemmas head on, speaking out when unethical actions, concepts or processes are occurring, or

-displaying a passion for ethics in the main.

Counteraction of ethics:

The modernised push for social or societal delineation of an individual is antithetic to the descriptions just provided.

It creates:

-inner chaos,

-constant questioning of oneself,

-self-loathing, and

-damaged self-identity.

SELF-NURTURED TRAITS

> One does not have to favour positive psychology to naturally nurture oneself, and one's particularly positive characteristics.

The desire to increase awareness of, enhance, or regularly utilise self-nurtured traits may emerge as a result of:

-an epiphany following a major life crisis/event

-(occur) upon reflection of age, life development stage, circumstance, or challenges set before you

-what works for the individual

-familial and interpersonal relationship influences

-injustices

-betrayal

-anxieties

-survival tactics (self-protection for instance)

-psychological damage, or traumatic experience/s.

Or, all of these can play a part.

<h1 style="text-align:center"><u>ASSESSMENT of (PERSONALITY or) PERSONALITY and ATTITUDINAL TRAITS:</u></h1>

There are many different reasons for the administration of personality tests, assessments and measures (so too, with attitudinal traits).
For instance:

"In the event of Self-disclosure, indicating anti-social/exploitative lifestyle behaviours, an assessment via a structured questionnaire, such as a personality test is recommended."
(11)

Personality traits' measures:

<u>**PRF-R: Personality Research Form- Revised; Jackson Personality Inventory-R (Revised) (3rd edition):**</u>

-examines *personality traits, covers various settings (employment recruitment, counselling, interpersonal, work, study, teams)*

-has multiple forms

-16-20 items

-measures harm avoidance; aggression; nurturance; infrequency; impulsivity, and so forth (Form E).

(12)

<u>MBTI: Myers Briggs Type Indicator</u>

-assesses *16 different personality types via 4 personality scales*

-has multiple forms

-measures Extraversion-Introversion; Sensing-Intuition; Thinking-Feeling; Judging-Perceiving.

The most recent update is the 2019 online version.

(13)

<u>SHL OPQ: Saville & Holdsworth Ltd Occupational Personality Questionnaire</u>

-measurement for *job role testing, leadership skills, employment recruitment*

-20 minutes to administer

-can be undertaken on line

-trait based personality measure

-30 different languages/translations

-32 dimensions:

   -Relationships with people (sociability, influence, empathy);

   -Thinking style (structure, creating and change, analysis);

   -Feelings and Emotions (dynamism, emotions);

involves 20 key competencies (leading & deciding; supporting & cooperating; interacting & presenting; analyzing & interpreting; creating & conceptualizing; organizing & executing; adapting & coping; enterprising & performing)

-104 questions/statements in opq32i

-multiple versions: OPQ32'r'; OPQ32i; OPQ32n;

-'r' is the shortest (n= normative, i= ipsative, r=shorter ipsative).

(14)

<u>DISC test (Dominance; Influence; Steadiness; Compliance/Conscientious)</u>
<u>(model created by Marston)</u>

-assesses *actions and behaviors versus cognitions*

-used to assess for job recruitment, employees, work productivity

-task-focussed, and people focussed

-28 items

-12 minutes completion

-multiple choice questions

-no right or wrong answers

-online testing.

(15)

<u>DSM-5- (and TR) recommended:</u>

PID-5-BF (The personality inventory for DSM-5- Brief form
-Adult);

PID-5 (the personality inventory for DSM-5- Adult) (9);

PID-5-IRF (the personality inventory for DSM-5- informant form- adult).

Also with relevance is:

Cattell's Sixteen Personality Factor Questionnaire (16PF)- 5th (and 6th ed.). (16)

Minnesota Multi-Phasic Personality Inventory (MMPI-3). (17)

Attitudinal traits' measures:

"Dispositional attitudes should be related to other traits that predispose individuals to experience positive or negative affect (e.g., extraversion, optimism)...". (18)

<u>DAM: Dispositional Attitude Measure (sometimes referred to as DAS)</u>

-measures *positive and negative dispositional attitudes by use of stimuli*

-individual attitudes focus

-16 items.

 (18)

JSDS: the Judgemental Self-Doubt Scale

-measures *judgemental ability and level of confidence in ability to make correct judgements*

-19 items

-moral dilemmas are included in items.
(19)

NFC- Short form: Need for Cognition scale- Short form

-measures *level of engaging in and enjoyment of thinking*

-18 items.

(20)

Personal values:

SVS- Schwartz Value Survey:

-measures *the motivational goal of each value:*

-self-direction;

-stimulation;

-hedonism;

-achievement;

-power;

-security;

-conformity;

-tradition;

-benevolence;

-universalism

-56-57 items total (combined from 2 scales)

-also cross-culturally relevant.
(1)

<u>DSM-5-TR AND ICD-11 RELATED PERSONALITY DISORDERS</u>

*The following personality disorders affect full awareness of one's inner self,
and can promote negative attitudinal traits.*

DSM-5-TR Personality disorders:

Narcissistic Personality disorder:

-identity: self-definition (as well as self-esteem) is determined by others

-self-direction: often incapable of self-awareness (motivations); self-concept is derived
 from self-entitlement

-empathy: is based on how others affect oneself; compromised ability to relate to the
 feelings and needs of other persons.

Borderline Personality disorder:

-identity: unstable sense of self (disturbance of identity); enduring feelings of emptiness;
 and become dissociative as a response to duress

-self-direction: "instability in goals, aspirations, values and career plans" (9)

-empathy: focussed on self and the negative effects of others upon oneself.

Anti-social Personality disorder:

-identity: "egocentrism; self-esteem derived from personal gain, power, or pleasure." (9)

-self-direction: ethical behavior and personal standards are compromised to the point of illegality; focus is always on satiating one's needs only

-empathy: "lack of concern for feelings, needs, or suffering of others; lack of remorse after hurting or mistreating another". (9)

It is proposed that people diagnosed with personality disorders, such as **Dependent Personality disorder**, also have cognitions and behaviors synonymous with identity disturbance, and self-direction:

For instance:

-inability to be alone;

-cannot function without others' support;

-feeling incapable of taking care of themselves;

-difficulties with decision-making;

-attachment issues (fear of abandonment);

-avoidance in taking personal responsibility.

ICD-11 Personality disorders:

Diagnosis of personality disorders via the **ICD-11** is used via a broader model, but is consistent with the alternative DSM-5 model for personality disorders.

That is:

-Personality difficulty, is assessed as either: mild; moderate; or severe personality disorder.

-Thence, identification of prominent traits, which affect personality functioning: negative affectivity; detachment; dissociality; disinhibition; anankastia (9)(a).

-In addition, there is a borderline pattern qualifier, though it is optional for inclusion.

For instance: severe personality disorder, with borderline pattern, with detachment, dissociality, and disinhibition.

DEVELOPMENTAL PSYCHOLOGY EFFECTS

-nurture and nature

-genetics naturally contribute to the formation of personality

-however both nature, and nurture, influence personality and attitudinal traits.

Some Nurture influencers involve:

-parental and social interactivity,

-childhood/upbringing,

-cultural environment, and

-experiences.

These enhance or minimise attitudinal leanings within social, political, and human relations, (for instance) domains.

-abuse, neglect, in childhood and the ramafications which force changes to innate personality and thus attitudinal traits, can exist in multiple circumstances

-stages of moral development

There are 3 primary levels, and multiple stages of moral development:

-preconventional: punishment/ obedience; rewards; and, needs seeking

-conventional: conformity to social rules; good boy/nice girl; law and order

-post-conventional: principled level; social contract; universal ethical principles.

Age does not necessarily determine at which stage one's moral development is situated.

There are many adult individuals, in all areas of life and work, who do not reach the full post-conventional level.

This is for a variety of reasons, and often can be a result of personality disorders, or deficits. For others, though they may appear to be stuck at a juvenile stage of moral development, they are actually fully aware of (and intrinsically comprehend) the post-conventional stages, but choose to reject adherence to the final stages on attitudinal, and personality predisposition, grounds.

-delayed developmental norms and impact on functioning in adulthood

This incorporates:

-cognitive

-communication

-motor

-socioemotional

-adaptive skills.

> **-learning disorders, dyslexia, and categorisation in school systems as 'abnormal', 'socially dysfunctional', or 'needy' (and, as handled inappropriately)**

Have the following effects:

-impact on identity formation

-crushing of self-esteem

-determines life-long decision making about significant: life and relationship choices

-can negatively compromise all 'normal' life functioning processes

-disadvantages, traumatises, and derogates, the individual as a result of labelling, abuse, neglect, and derision.

> **-heavy indoctrination of anarchic identity principles**

-"People differ in their fundamental, individual tendencies, such as their conception of self, which might result in the emergence of diverse perceptions of group cohesion"
(2)

-can create delay or compromisation in self-identity development

-behaviors, cognitions and decision-making which are at loggerheads with personal values and intuition.

> **-extreme socialist ideologies and crisis of confusion regarding pre-adolescent attitudinal trait development**

-aggression: impulsive, violent, extreme negative emotions

-anger: (likewise with aggression) hostile cognitions, and rumination about perceived unfair treatment, poor coping mechanisms, and hyper-arousal physiologically

-sociopathy (anti-social personality disorder): "manipulativeness, deceitfulness, hostility, and with psychopathy: high levels of attention-seeking".

(21)

TRAITS and EXPECTATIONS of HEALTHCARE PROFESSIONALS

The points made below are not extrapolated to define the right and wrong expectations made by society, patients, caregivers, or healthcare leaders, or necessarily what should exist (or not exist) within a given healthcare professional.

It is a description of some of the common traits, and expectations, of healthcare service providers.

resilience

"reasonable resilience incorporates multiple inner resources which require nurturing and maturing over time.

For instance:

-psychological resilience: withstanding disappointments, and recognising their impermanency

-emotional resilience: being able to temper extreme emotions in the face of adversity

-physical resilience: endurance with- boundaries and acceptable- limits

-cognitive resilience: comprehending, and deciphering, truth from fiction."

(22)

strength of character

-truthfulness

-honesty

-fairness

-compassion

-ethical

-perseverance

-fortitude

-capacity for self-regulation

-multi-tasks without given to stressors.

innately assertive

-assertiveness can sometimes be cultivated by learned techniques

-personality and attitudinal traits, however, do pre-determine one's propensity for reacting
 in a confident, assured way to conflict, compromisation of rights, and so forth

-to exemplify the necessity of assertiveness: "To create a feeling of foreboding, fearfulness,
and terror, in a healthcare (or other), worker paralyses, shocks, and overwhelms. When it
moves to the physical, compliance is usually the reaction. However, inaction and
surrender, usually exacerbates the bully further." (23)

-with notable knowledge, and experience, in the healthcare field, comes the expectation from management through to patients, of the healthcare worker's power of intuition

-often overestimated, there is an expectation that the healthcare professional will be able to intuit for diagnosis or correct treatment regimens without being provided with the full clinical information

-nevertheless, many healthcare workers rely on their intuition in circumstances that are blurred

-it is a vulnerable quality, and part of the inner self. Exhaustion, or feeling over-worked, can easily cause one to question their intuition, and elicit second-guessed response behaviors.

-responsibility knows no bounds in healthcare

-the concept of being, and behaving, in a responsible way differs

-effective responsibility comes from an inner sensibility, a solid ethical framework, and a commitment to quality and safety for patients, colleagues, and the healthcare system.

-this does not just pertain to newly graduated healthcare professional students nor is it necessarily age, experience, or status, related

-from best practice based care pathways, and digital communication operations, to efficient use of these models, and healthcare professions' regulatory framework, maturity of thought is evidently not a concept contained to the individual healthcare worker.

Nevertheless, on an individual healthcare professional basis the following related behaviors are relevant:

-observance of patient safety culture

-information driven collegial networking, as per needed

-self-honesty, seeking advice when unsure clinically

-cognitive and emotional processing contributing to positive work culture.

So too, maturity of thought cognitions:

-patient centered mentality

-belief in self, and professional prowess

-rational thinking

-confidence in abilities

-emotional stability: in not being governed by ego, sensitivities, or easily taking offence.

Cognitive, emotional, and behavioral, flexibility and adaptability is considered an overall necessity.

hardiness

Hardiness naturally and vastly differs from hardness.

Hardiness is similar to resilience, it is a capability of enduring challenging conditions.

It is typically defined as:

-coping, control and challenge

-the capacity to respond and handle stressors

-without surrendering to:

   -feelings of powerlessness

   -fatigue

and to control one's emotional reactions accordingly:

-exemplary level of commitment

-active coping strategies as utilised continuously and effectively.

unbreakable

-inability to weaken the healthcare workers' stance against wrongdoings

-durability in the face of inordinate healthcare challenges

-can withstand torment, bullying, overworking, long shifts, and conflict

-regardless of issues in one's private life, work productivity, efficiency, safety and quality
levels, remain of best practice standards.

immune

-this can be understood in 2 forms:

    -immunity to emotional impacts of constantly witnessing suffering; and

    -immunity from being drawn into, or causing, medical error- along with blameworthiness.

adaptable

-can adjust work styles, emotions, cognitions and behaviors easily when faced with
changes to work environment, protocols, procedures, and work duties

-concomitant coping styles can be changed to facilitate required adaptability

-psychological flexibility is a key component of coping in an adaptable way.

all-inclusive, all-encompassing

-team-work orientated, although capable of independent thought and action

-all intradisciplinary (and interdisciplinary) team members are in harmony with each other

-ideally: patient, caregivers, interdisciplinary healthcare professional team members, including physicians, nurses, and allied healthcare workers work together in a patient-centered way

-diagnostic and treatment initiatives (and care planning) are undertaken, formulated, and reviewed, from a patient safety and quality of healthcare perspective

-positive attributes of the healthcare professional are continuously improving to incorporate newest medical research initiatives

-healthcare workers, facility, and system functionality, is: frequently reviewed to prevent critical incidents, other patient harm, and observes adherence to mandatory healthcare obligations.

ABBREVIATIONS

16PF: Cattell's Sixteen Personality Factor Questionnaire

DAM/DAS: Dispositional Attitude Measure

DISC: Dominance; Influence; Steadiness; Compliance/Conscientious

DSM-5-TR: Diagnostic and Statistics Manual for Mental Disorders-5th Edition- Text
Revision

FFM: Five Factor Model

HEXACO: Honesty-Humility; Emotionality; eXtraversion; Agreeableness (vs Anger);
Conscientiousness; Openness to Experience

JSDS: Judgemental Self-Doubt Scale

MBTI: Myers Briggs Type Indicator

MMPI-3: Minnesota Multi-Phasic Personality Inventory-3

NFC-Short form: Need for Cognition Scale- Short form

OCEAN: Openness to experience; Conscientiousness; Extraversion;
Agreeableness; Neuroticism

PID-5: The personality inventory for DSM-5- Adult)

PID-5-BF: The personality inventory for DSM-5- Brief form-Adult

PID-5-IRF: The personality inventory for DSM-5- informant form- adult

PRF-R: Personality Research Form- Revised

SHL- OPQ: Saville & Holdsworth Ltd Occupational Personality Questionnaire

SHL-OPQ32i: ipsative

SHL-OPQ32n: normative

SHL-OPQ32r: shorter ipsative

SVS: Schwartz Value Survey

1/ What are the 10 basic human values?

2/ Please define 'intuition'.

3/ Does 'rationalization' play a part in intuition?

4/ Which factors enhance belief in self?

5/ Name 3 elements involved in personality characteristics.

6/ How can emotional content be more easily recognised?

7/ How can challenges be beneficial to the inner self?

8/ Please define 'identity'.

9/ Describe a personal experience involving innate reactions to specific circumstances.

10/ 'True self' is described as:

   a) me, myself, and I

   b) assured presence of mind

   c) often differs from social self

   d) all of the above.

11/ Add 2 factors which you consider additionally contribute to universal vulnerabilities.

12/ Does self-respect affect self-esteem. If so, in which ways?

13/ Detail 2 other factors which effect self-esteem levels.

14/ What is your understanding of the 'ideal self' and 'the real self'?

15/ What do you consider to be most important in life?

16/ Which other elements of self-esteem dovetail with self-concept?

17/ Name the term which represents the pinnacle of achievement in self-growth.

18/ Is unconditional acceptance a factor relating to the inner self. If so, please extrapolate.

19/ What is your opinion of the featured formulaic content. Add further specifics relevant to your own knowledge and experience.

20/ Describe 'self-belief'.

21/ Which elements of the inner self will especially prevail in the face of challenge to one's self-confidence?

22/ How is mental fitness beneficial?

23/ What is your understanding of emotional intelligence?

24/ Complete the sentence: 'problem solving abilities are part of......'

25/ What is concomitant with 'self-regulation'?

26/ Explain the difference between 'self-efficacy' and 'self-esteem'.

27/ In your opinion, in which ways are you unique?

28/ Your inner core remains throughout one's lifetime, regardless of perceptions that it is:

    a) irreparable

    b) destroyed

    c) intangible

    d) all of the above.

29/ Explain the main differences between cardinal; central; and, secondary, traits.

30/ Which personality trait focussed scholar placed importance upon analysis of prejudice and religion?

31/ How can immature religion be described?

32/ Please define 'attitude'.

33/ What is the 'FFM'?

34/ Provide 2 differences between the FFM and the HEXACO model.

35/ In which scale (of the HEXACO model) does 'prudence' belong?

36/ What is the difference between 'extraversion' and 'extroversion'?

37/ Describe social boldness.

38/ Which term applies to: being co-operative with ability to compromise?

39/ Emotionality consists of:

      a) dependence

      b) fearfulness

      c) anger

      d) a) and b)

40/ In your opinion, how necessary is 'altruism'?

41/ What are the 3 main components of the Dark triad personality traits?

42/ In which Dark triad personality does moral corruption play a part?

43/ Provide 3 core traits of narcissism.

44/ Anti-social personality, sociopathy, and psychopathy are often terms used interchangeably. What in your opinion, are the defining features of 'psychopathy versus sociopathy'?

45/ What is the polar opposite to detachment? Please discuss.

46/ Which particular traits are influential upon attitudes/attitudinal traits?

47/ Attitudinal traits involve the:

      a) affective

      b) behavioral

      c) cognitive

      d) all of the above.

48/ Complete the sentence: 'change is ripe, where there exists.......'

49/ What are 3 modes of change which can contribute to attitudinal traits?

50/ Which individual character traits may provide resistance to attitudinal influences?

51/ What is the meaning of subterfuge in compliance with attitudinal change?

52/ Detail the Five hazardous attitudes.

53/ How is knowledge of the Five hazardous attitudes relevant to healthcare?

54/ What is your understanding of 'root cause analysis'?

55/ Upon which factors does value of ethics depend?

56/ Have you ever spoken out against unethical action/s? Please describe.

57/ What can the modernised push for social acquiescence create?

58/ What are some of the reasons for inspired self-nurturing of one's traits?

59/ Name 3 personality traits' measures, and provide details.

60/ In which measure does assessment of 'sensing-intuition' feature?

61/ What is the DISC?

62/ What is the MMPI-3?

63/ Which type of measure is the JSDS?

64/ What does the NFC measure?

65/ Please name a personal values measure.

66/ From recall, select one DSM-5 (and 5-TR) based personality disorder. Provide a description of identity, self-direction, and empathy.

67/ Describe Dependent personality disorder symptomatology.

68/ In which ways does ICD-11's approach to personality disorders differ?

69/ Think about someone who knows you, have met, or have knowledge of, who may present with symptoms consistent with a personality disorder. Provide an ICD-11 based description of them.

70/ What are the 3 primary levels of moral development?

71/ Choose 1 of the 3 levels of moral development and name the stages involved.

72/ How can negative categorization in the school system impact an individual- developmentally?

73/ What possible effects can come of heavy indoctrination (anarchically)?

74/ Provide the differences between 'anger' and 'aggression'.

75/ Define 'resilience'.

76/ What, in your opinion, are the primary personality and attitudinal traits expected of healthcare professionals?

77/ What is meant by 'perseverance'?

78/ Explain what may occur as a result of delayed assertiveness in relation to bullying.

79/ Which factors can influence a healthcare worker questioning their own intuition?

80/ Please describe the underpinnings of 'effective responsibility'.

81/ Maturity of thought is not necessarily age-related. What are the components of such?

82/ Hardiness is typically defined as:

   a) coping

   b) challenge

   c) control

   d) all of the above

83/ Is being perceived to be 'unbreakable' a positive or negative experience? Please discuss.

84/ How are healthcare professionals considered as 'immune'?

85/ How can one otherwise term 'psychological flexibility'?

86/ What is meant by being 'all inclusive, all encompassing'?

REFERENCES

(1) Schwartz, S.H. (2012), An overview of Schwartz theory of basic values, Online Readings in Psychology and Culture, 2(1).

(2) Paunova, M. & Li-Ying, J. (2023), Original article: Interactive effects of self-concept and social context on perceived cohesion in intensive care nursing, Applied Psychology, Vol.72(1), 2023, 268-296.

(3) Allport, G.W. (1935), Attitudes, in C.M. Murchison (Ed.). Handbook of social psychology, M.A.: Clark University Press, p.810.

(4) Allport, G.W. (1950), The individual and his religion, N.Y.: Mcmillan, p.viii.

(5) Allport, G.W. (1950), The individual and his religion: a psychological interpretation, Toronto:macmillan, p.72.

(6) McCrae, R.R., & Costa Jr, P.T. (2008), the five factor theory of personality . In O.P. John, R.W. Robins, & L.A. Pervin (Eds.), Handbook of Personality: Theory and Research (3rd ed.), N.Y.: Guildford Press, pp. 159-181.

(7) Lee, K & Ashton, M.C., 2009, The Hexaco Personality Inventory- Revised: A Measure of the Six Major Dimensions of Personality in www.hexaco.org

(8) Paulhus, D.L. & Williams, K.M. (2002), The dark triad of personality: Narcissism, machiavellianism and psychopathy, Journal of Research in Personality, 36 (6), 556-563.

(9)American Psychiatric Association (2022), Diagnostic and Statistical Manual of Mental Disorders, 5 th ed. Text Revision: DSM-5-TR. Washington, D.C.: American Psychiatric Association Publishing, pp. 884; 886; 894; 899-901.

(9) (a) World Health Organization (2019), International Statistical Classification of Diseases and Related Health Problems, 11th ed,; ICD-11.

(10) Federal Aviation Administration (2009), Risk management handbook, Washington, DC: Government Printing Office, pp. 2-5.

(11) Tophus, M.D. (2022), Who is this colleague?: Dangers of the healthcare profession, and beyond. An interview guide for recruitment, performance appraisal and post-adverse events, Germany: Hilphma Publications, p.46.

(12) Jackson, D.N. (1984), Personality Research Form manual (3rd ed.), Port Huron: Sigma Assessment Systems.

(13) Myers & Briggs Foundation (2022), MBTI, www.myersbriggs.org

(14) Saville & Holdsworth Ltd. (2022), SHL Occupational Personality Questionnaire (OPQ), www.shl.com

(15) Marston, W.M. (1928), Emotions of normal people, London/N.Y.: Harcourt, Brace & Co.

(16) Cattell, H.B. & Shuerger, J.M. (2003), Essentials of 16PF assessment, Hoboken, N.J.: John Wiley.

(17) Ben-Porath, Y.S. & Tellegen, A. (2020), The Minnesota Multiphasic Personality Inventory-3: Manual for administration, scoring, and interpretation. University of Minnesota Press.

(18) Hepler, J. & Albarracin, D., (2013), Attitudes without objects: Evidence for a dispositional attitude, its measurement, and its consequences, J Pers. Soc. Psychol., 2013 jun; 104(6): 1060-1076.

(19) Mirels, H.L., Greblo, P. & Dean, J.B. (2002), Judgemental self-doubt: Beliefs about one's judgemental prowess, Personality and Individual Differences, 33, 741-758.

(20) Cacciopo, J.T., Petty, R.E, & Kao, C.F. (1984), The efficient assessment of need for cognition, Journal of Personality Assessment, 48, 306-307.

(21) Tophus, M.D. (2023), The controversy of the remorseless and unempathic healthcare worker, Germany: Hilphma Publications, p.21.

(22) Tophus, M.D. (2022), Reasonable resilience in workplaces and healthcare work, Germany: Hilphma Publications, pp.16-17.

(23) Tophus, M.D. (2022), The A to Z of Workplace Bullying: For the Healthcare Professional and Beyond, Germany: Hilphma Publications, p.27.

extrovert 31
facilitate 55
facility 56
factor 30
factors 15; 22
fairness 25; 51
faith 21; 22
familial 35
fatigue 54
fear 12; 24
fearfulness 24; 51
fears 14
feeling 51
feeling/s 8; 10; 11; 12; 38; 43; 44; 54
FFM 22; 57
fiction 50
five factor 28
five hazardous attitudes 31
flexibility 24; 53; 55
focus 19; 23
foreboding 51
forgivingness 24
formation 48
forms 37; 38
formulated 56
fortitude 51
framework 52
frequency 11
Freud 20
function 44
functionality 56
functioning 17; 45; 47
fundamental 48
furthering 17
genetics 46
gentleness 24
goal/s 15; 16; 18; 32; 41; 43
good boy 47
graduated 52
grandiose 26
greed 20; 25
group 48
handled 48
happiness 12
hardiness 54
harm avoidance 37
harmony 55
healthcare 22; 31; 32; 33; 50; 51; 52; 54; 56
healthcare field 52